THE ART OF AGING

Mabel Monks

THE ART OF AGING

MABEL MONKS

Foreword by

MARILYN MONKS PAGE

ABOUT THE AUTHOR

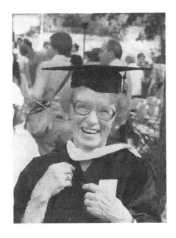

Mabel Monks was born and grew up in Worcester, MA. She lived and raised her five children in the home in which she was born on the top of Heard Street Hill just up from Hadwen Park. She was a late bloomer. In her sixties, she got her driving license. That was quite a milestone. And after seeing that senior citizens could attend Clark University for free, at age sixty-eight, she enrolled in classes; after several years as a co-ed, she graduated summa cum laude in humanities when she was seventy-two years old. At age seventy-eight, Mabel became a widow and lived for the next ten years independently, serving as a docent for the Worcester Antiquarian Society, giving lectures on the architecture of Worcester to middle-school children, being active in her church, and traveling with Elder Hostel (now Road Scholar). When she was eighty-eight, she sold the home she had lived in since birth, bought an apartment in a retirement home in York, Maine, and has lived independently, meaningfully, and actively in her apartment since that time. Mabel is ninety-nine years old.

Contact Mabel Monks and Marilyn Monks Page at www.marilynmonkspage.com

Mabel Monks

Pollywog Pond Press, a division of Warrington Press

San Francisco, CA

Printed in the United States of America

ISBN-10: 0-692-22980-9
ISBN-13: 978-0-692-22980-4

Contents

Foreword

We all know about hoarders. I would be the opposite of a hoarder. I love to get rid of things. And so I was cleaning out my office closet and feeling freer and freer as I tossed one thing after another into the trash bag. Then I found a paper on aging that Grandma had written, while she was a senior-citizen graduate student at Worcester State College, two years after she had graduated from Clark University in Worcester, MA. Grandma is not my grandmother; she is my mother. But I have become so used to calling her Grandma around my children and nieces and nephews, that that is now what I call her when I am talking about her.

This paper represented a lot of work on Grandma's part . It also was a clear treatise on how one person thought about getting older. I couldn't throw away such a valuable piece of history. I thought about how important and meaningful this could be to other people and to her family, especially her grandchildren and great-grandchildren. Never mind her grandchildren and great-grandchildren, her children are now close to or past the age Grandma was when she wrote it. It might be a bible of sorts for them.

What better way to share this with the world than to convert it into a book. And so, here it is—Grandma's story about how she thought about aging as well as what she thought about while she was aging. This is a story about how experiences in her life impacted how she thought and how those experiences sustained her and propelled her forward as she aged.

Enjoy the journey along with Grandma.

Marilyn Monks Page, author of *Out-of-School Tales of a Reluctant Educator* at http://www.amazon.com

Introduction

Aging, the natural process which begins at birth and passes through the stages of life—infancy, childhood, youth, adulthood, and finally to old age—is living. If aging stops, life is over. The way we look at aging and living determines in large measure the kind of life that is in store for us. Aging is a different phenomenon for each individual, occurring in different ways and at different stages of a person's life. We go merrily along, living each day as it comes, not really thinking about aging, until, almost overnight, we realize that much time has passed, and there is evidence that we are truly growing older.

The subject of aging and growing old has been contemplated and written about from the time of Euripides and Aristotle—who presented pessimistic views of old age—to Cicero, who—in his treatise, *On Old Age,*—was more optimistic about the later years of life. He said:

> *The fact is that old age is respectable just as long as it asserts itself, maintains its proper rights and is not enslaved to anyone. For as I admire a young man who has something of the old man in him, so do I an old one who has something of a young man. The man who aims at this may possibly become old in body—in mind he never will.*

Throughout the centuries, attitudes toward growing old have differed depending upon conditions under which people lived at any given time. In February, 1975, social historian, David Hackett Fischer, presented the Bland-Lee Lectures at Clark University in Worcester, MA. These lectures were the basis for his book, *Growing Old in America,* which puts into historical perspective attitudes about age relations through past centuries to the present time.

During the early years of the American colonies, leaders were chosen from the elders of the community. Religious teachings emphasized respect for the elderly. The Puritans felt that to survive to old age showed God's approval and was God's reward for a life lived according to the accepted religious beliefs of the time. Fischer quotes Increase Mather who said, "There is something of the image of God in age." It was presumed that old men knew more than younger ones and that aged persons were the fittest to be trusted with the offices of honor in the community.

Following the Revolutionary War, the attitudes toward the aged began to change. Old age became more common; people were living longer. At the same time, the old were regarded with increasing contempt. Whereas the clergy venerated age, the literature reflected opposing opinions. Thoreau, at the age of thirty, expressed his contempt for all those older than he when he said:

Age is no better, hardly so well, qualified for an instructor as youth, for it has not profited so much as it has lost. One may almost doubt if the wisest man has learned anything of absolute value by living. Practically, the old have no very important advice to give the young, their experience has been so partial, and their lives have been such miserable failures, for private reasons, as they must believe; and it may be that they have some faith left which belies that experience, and they are only less young than they were.

Hawthorne, in the introduction to *The Scarlet Letter*, says:

The white locks of age were sometimes found to be the thatch of an intellectual tenement in good repair. But, as respects the majority of my corps of veterans, there will be no wrong done, if I characterize them generally as a set of wearisome old souls, who had gathered nothing worth preservation from their varied experience of life.

These attitudes were the foundation for the present day concentration on a youth-oriented society.

Longfellow has summarized, in a way, the attitudes about aging in his poem, *Morituri Salutamus,* (the gladiator's motto—*We who are about to die salute you*). It was written on the occasion of his fiftieth reunion at Bowdoin College and concludes with an inspiring view of growing older:

The Art of Aging

Whatever poet, orator, or sage
May say of it, old age is still old age,
It is the waning, not the crescent moon;
The dusk of evening, not the blaze of noon;
It is not strength, but weakness; not desire,
But its surcease; not the fierce heat of fire,
The burning and consuming element,
But that of ashes and of embers spent,
In which some living sparks we still discern,
Enough to warm, but not enough to burn.

What then? Shall we sit idly down and say
The night hath come; it is no longer day?
The night hath not yet come; we are not quite
Cut off from labor by the failing light;
Something remains for us to do or dare;
Even the oldest tree some fruit may bear;
Not the Oedipus Coloneus, or Greek Ode,
Or tales of pilgrims that one morning rode
Out of the gateway of the Tabard Inn,
But other something, would we but begin;
For age is opportunity no less
Than youth itself, though in another dress,
And as the evening twilight fades away
The sky is filled with stars, invisible by day.

Mabel Monks

Conversation 1

"How old are you, Grandma?" Sarah asks as we walk along the high road overlooking the ocean.

"How old do you think I am?" I ask in reply.

Then the guessing game begins. "Are you ninety?" they ask.

"Not quite," I answer, and the three little girls continue the guessing—fifty, eighty, seventy-five—until they are close enough to the truth.

Then they exclaim, "That's very old, isn't it?"

Grandparents must, indeed, appear very old to seven and eight-year-olds.

"Did you come to Maine when you were a little girl?"

"When I was as old as you are, we didn't have a car, so we stayed in Worcester. Sometimes we took a train trip to see my grandparents."

"What is it like to ride on a train?" Sarah asks.

We talk about trains and how exciting it was to wait in the big station, crowded with people, and to listen for the trainmaster to announce that our train was coming; how we would hurry to the platform, wait for people to get off, and climb up the high steps into the train. The whistle would blow, the engine would chug a couple of times, and we would be on our way.

Sarah thinks it would be fun to ride on a train and Jeannie and Carrie tell her about their train rides to Chicago and Florida. We clamber over the rocks near the lighthouse and sit near the water to watch the waves smashing against the shore.

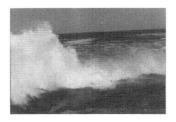 "Sarah, what are you going to be when you grow up?" I ask.

"Oh, I would like to be a ballet dancer, so I could be in the Nutcracker," she says.

The others have answers too. Jeannie—maybe a teacher like her mother. Carrie—well, she might like to be a nurse. Tomorrow their ideas will change. Soon they will say, "When I am old enough …, or "I'll be glad when I am old enough to do what grown-ups do—drive a car, get a job, have my own money, wear make-up. They can't wait to grow older. The future appears bright and exciting.

I am at the other end of the life line. I no longer anticipate with eagerness the passing of years. Rather, I relish each new day that is given to me.

The girls are restless—anxious to move on. "Let's go over to the frog pond," they say. We leave behind the ocean and the lighthouse. Our conversation about growing older already forgotten as they listen for the conversation of the frogs.

I contemplate the conversation with my young grand-daughters and wonder at the difference in attitudes about growing older. Youth looks eagerly to the future, anticipating the added years; growing older is a great adventure. Older people wish to recapture their youth or at least slow down the passage of time.

Why do we lose enthusiasm for the future as we grow older? Is it the nature of man that enthusiasm for life wanes or is it the result of the stereotypical conditioning people are exposed to during their lifetime?

When retirement arrives, it is the time to consider how to live the following years. Will we retreat into a life of inactivity, boredom, and emphasis on the glories of the past or will we look ahead with anticipation to the coming years and finding original ways to create a meaningful and fulfilling life?

As youth looks ahead to the unknown years, so we, too, should approach our later years with renewed vitality and hope for good times ahead as we pass the second turning point in our lives.

The Second Turning Point

In his book, *Learning to Grow Old,* Dr. Paul Tournier, a Swiss physician, speaks about the turning points in our lives. He defines one as the passage from childhood to adulthood and the second as the passage from adulthood to old age. He declares:

> *The second turning point is in no sense a*
> *step backward. It is an advance into new*
> *fulfillment. We should look upon our*
> *later years as a time to rediscover our*
> *spontaneity and originality*—a time to
> advance to a more complete fulfillment of
> one's self.

I have reached the magical age—the second turning point. What am I going to do about it? The home population has reduced over the past few years from seven to two with a comparable reduction in the laundry, meals, beds to make, and the number of people sharing in the use of the one family car. Now is the perfect time to do all the things that I have been waiting for years to try or finish— now I can complete the half-finished projects.

The experts believe that retirement activities should be planned long before the onset of the golden years. However, more often than not, it doesn't happen that way. Only a super person could consciously take time to map out a regimen of daily activities for the unknown magical years, when twenty-four hour days are not enough to take care of a growing family. Unconsciously, perhaps, I was preparing for my later years when I developed leisure activities and skills in my limited spare time. Some of these activities have carried over to play a rewarding part in my life. Playing the piano, which when I had to practice every day was a tedious chore, has become a source of great enjoyment for me.

However, life has changed. There is no longer even a good reason to get up at any special time. If I am wise, now is the time to follow Tournier's advice and rediscover spontaneity and originality and advance to a more complete fulfillment of myself.

Consider these qualities for a moment. Spontaneity. If I understand what it means, it is an attribute which has never come easily to me. The dictionary defines it as *the quality of proceeding or acting from native feeling, proneness, or temperament without constraint or external force.*

Perhaps as a child I acted more spontaneously, although my memory tells me that I have always felt constraints placed upon me to act according to the accepted norms—to meet the expectations of others. It is only now, in these later years, that I feel a growing need to do what I want to do, answer to my own ideas. It has never been a hardship for me to follow others' ideas and plans. There was always plenty of time ahead for what I would really like to do. Now the time is getting shorter and there are so many new experiences I would like to explore. A change is taking place and somehow I'm finding a way to take advantage of opportunities which are presented to me.

Emily's story presents ideas about spontaneity and initiative which appeal to me, ideas with which I can agree and which I hope to emulate.

Walls

The tour bus stopped before the small hotel overlooking the Rhine River, and for the fifteenth time in as many days, Emily followed Louise out of the bus and into the lobby to go through the registering routine—passports out, sign the book, receive the key.

"Passport," said the desk clerk in his clipped German accent. "Sign the book; room 11," and he slapped the key on the desk top.

They picked up their suitcases and struggled into the tiny elevator which could carry a maximum of two people and their luggage. It lifted slowly to the first floor. They pushed the bags into the corridor and found their room just around the corner.

Emily sank into the nearest chair and kicked off her shoes. She was tired. Every part of her feet ached in spite of the housemaid's shoes she wore. Her knees were almost locked in a bent position from climbing the steps of every museum and cathedral in every city along the route. The volumes of history and related information her mind had consumed in the past two weeks, along with the constant chatter of other tourists as the bus traversed the landscape between stops, had her mind doing tumble-saults.

It had been a good trip so far—France, Italy, and Austria—snow-topped Alps silhouetted against bright, blue sky, deep lakes, dark green pine forests. The cities, alive with people and traffic rushing together in the streets, barely escaping collisions—the usual tourist sights. But she needed to rest and Louise was babbling on about the great show they would see after a fabulous dinner in a small restaurant, near the cathedral, where the waiters wore long blue aprons as they carried six over-flowing steins, in each hand, to the eager customers.

Emily was not going. Why did she let other people make plans for her? Louise did it all the time. She was a good friend and fun to be with, but insisted on making all the plans, and Emily followed blindly along.

"Louise," she said, "I'm not going. A train leaves at eleven tonight for Berlin and I'm going to be on it. I can rest on the train." Louise was speechless as she watched Emily gather a few clothes in her bag and stretch out on the bed until it was time to leave.

It was 11 p.m. by the trainmaster's clock above platform #4 and the flashing sign announced that the train from Passau to Berlin was due in eight minutes. Emily opened her bag once again to be sure her ticket and passport were safe and held tightly to her suitcase. She was nervous. Would she be able to manage on her own? She wasn't sure, but for once in her life, she was going to ignore her fears and timidness and enjoy herself.

She glanced at the people waiting with her. Some seemed very relaxed; some men were reading the evening paper; a young girl with a back-pack was leaning against the wall reading a book. Others were just waiting. There were families with small children and weary parents resting on their luggage—bulging boxes tied with thick twine, old-fashioned wicker suitcases, and string bags holding the necessities for the trip. A man dashed up the stairs, grabbed the hand rail of the last car of a departing train, and scrambled aboard. Luggage wagons hurried up and down the platform.

One man, dressed in a dark grey, pinstriped suit was pacing back and forth. He seemed as nervous as she was. He lit cigarette after cigarette, never finishing one before stamping it out and lighting another; alternately he picked up and put down his small bag, checked his watch, and paced some more. Then he was gone, disappearing into the crowd.

An announcement blared from the loud speaker. Emily couldn't understand it. Was it about her train? She would have to watch closely as the trains arrived. One was coming. The wheels screeched against the tracks and the train for Berlin stopped in front of her. Doors flung open, the steps dropped, and the passengers poured out onto the platform.

Two long seats, covered in a paisley-patterned velvet, faced each other in the compartment. It was hot and smelled of stale tobacco smoke. She lifted her bag onto the iron rack overhead and settled into a comfortable position on the seat near the window.

As the whistle sounded for the train to leave, the door opened and a young man, probably about thirty, entered, tossed his bag onto the rack, and sat opposite her. With a quick nod for a greeting, he opened his book as if dismissing any thought of a conversation. He looked familiar. Yes, it was the restless young man she had watched on the platform.

The train picked up speed. Stations flashed past—Dortmund, Hannover—the whistle blowing at each one. By now, the young man had stretched out on the seat and was sleeping fitfully. The smooth rhythm of the train and the heat in the compartment made her sleepy, too. She covered herself with her raincoat and dozed against the seat.

Suddenly, the train came to a quick, jolting stop. From the window she saw uniformed soldiers on the platform preparing to board the train. The young man was awake, too.

"Why have we stopped here?" she asked anxiously. "And what do the soldiers want?"

He hesitated a few seconds, and then, almost bitterly it seemed, he replied. "We are at the border—the *Wall*—the place where free men are separated from those whose freedoms are restricted. It is this wall which divides families. The guards will ask for passports. They will inspect the luggage. Look out the window now and you will see men examining the train."

He was right. Men, wearing heavy, long, grey coats and army-type boots, were kneeling beside the train, pushing large, long-handled mirrors beneath the cars to see if anything or anyone was concealed there.

A sharp, staccato rap at the door and two stern, unsmiling soldiers confronted them. In clipped, guttural German, one asked for passports. They inspected the luggage and left, taking the passports with them. When would they return them, she wondered.

This was East Germany now. It was a rough ride. The tracks were uneven and the car swayed and bumped along more slowly than before. Emily was wide awake after the excitement of the past hour, even though it was only three o'clock in the morning and three hours away from Berlin.

The young man, too, was awake and staring out into the blackness. He still seemed disturbed. Maybe she should speak to him. She introduced herself and asked where he was from. Again he hesitated before replying, as if collecting his thoughts.

"My name is Karl Schmidt and I live in Canada. I was born in Berlin and I am going back for the first time since the war. I was a child then, about ten years old. I remember this city as it was. What fun we had playing football in the fields; running in familiar streets; and then returning, after playing, to the small apartment of my parents."

"Then came the terror of the war," he continued. "My family was separated when the city was divided. My mother and I were in the Western part. My father was still serving in the army in the East. We never saw him again. He is buried someplace there. For the first time, the authorities will allow people from the West to visit their families in the Eastern zone. It will not be the same, but I must go to see my relatives who are there." He turned again to the window and stared into the darkness.

Emily was disturbed. She had never met anyone who had lived through the experience of war as Karl had. Oh, she had felt the effects of the war at home—the food rationing, the inconvenience of coupons for meat, sugar and gasoline; the air-raid practices with the black-out shades pulled tight and lights out when the men donned their tin helmets and patrolled the streets until the all-clear signal sounded. But the war had not taken the men in her family to serve in the army. They worked in critical industry. She couldn't imagine what it would be like to be forcibly separated from her family. What grief and agony these people suffered!

The sky was lighter—almost daylight. Another sharp rap on the door and the soldiers entered with the passports. Karl moved restlessly, stood up, put Emily's suitcase on the seat beside her, picked up his own bag, and, as the train slowed into the station, with a quick *goodbye*, he left the compartment.

Emily congratulated herself. She was doing very well on her own. She found the hotel a short distance from the drab, cold station and treated herself to a leisurely breakfast of crisp rolls and hot coffee. There was time for a hot shower and an hour or so to relax before the bus left for East Berlin.

Check-point Charlie, as the grim, sinister barrier was called, where visitors entered East Berlin, loomed before them. A large sign, written in four languages, announced, *You are now leaving the American Sector.*

Border guards, dressed in drab, green uniforms and carrying rifles over their shoulders, goose-stepped along the top of the wall between the barbed-wire screens. Others peered through binoculars first in one direction and then in the other, monitoring every movement on the ground.

Heavy cement posts, set in a zigzag arrangement like a ski slalom, prevented cars from speeding to the West. There was the mirror technique again, this time under cars. Would anyone really try to escape by hanging between the wheels? Perhaps, if they were desperate enough. Car seats were removed. Luggage carriers were inspected and the contents spilled onto the ground and left for the owner to pick up.

Guards entered the bus. They opened bags to make sure no western literature was carried across the border. They scrutinized passports again; new tour guides came on board; and the bus continued.

13

This was not going to be a happy trip. Emily would rest, but her mind already was distressed by what she was seeing. The guide, speaking in understandable English, enthusiastically described and lauded the progress which had been made in rebuilding the city. Emily, at the same time, looked at the empty streets with traffic lights changing from red to green and no cars to obey them. The tiny, dim shops displayed a few utilitarian items, and rows of stark apartment houses lined the streets. Women, whose faces reflected the hardships they had endured and were still experiencing in their daily lives, walked along the sidewalks carrying worn shopping bags.

Emily thought of Karl Schmidt coming home to find his family. Was his father buried in the mass grave with thousands of other young men? What a waste all war was.

She had seen enough; in spite of the guide's glowing descriptions of buildings and monuments and of progress supposedly made, Emily was anxious to return to the free city of West Berlin.

Bright sunshine was streaming into the hotel room when Emily woke the next morning. She was rested and hungry. She relished again the fresh rolls and hot coffee. She was ready to start the return journey. The train passed fields, golden with ripe grain. Men and women were working together, tossing the grain into piles to be picked up by horse-drawn farm wagons. On through the large, smokey, industrial cities and then arrival in Cologne.

Emily was excited and refreshed. The trip was over and she was ready to rejoin the group. She had passed safely through two walls—the forbidding Check-Point Charlie and her own personal wall which had, for so many years, kept her under the domination of other people.

She was free.

One of the advantages of growing older is the ability, because of earlier experiences, to deal creatively with walls imposed by others, by ourselves, or by conditions of our everyday life—an ability to break away from past behavior and create new ways to overcome or to live happily within the restraints of these walls. We must conquer or adjust to walls throughout life from childhood to old age: walls of school, walls of work, walls of family responsibilities, walls of physical disabilities, walls of loneliness. These are only a few of the walls or restrictions which we encounter during a lifetime.

People respond differently to the restrictions of the walls of life. Some live quietly and without rebellion within all restrictions, while others are constantly battling against all confining elements in their lives. Neither extreme is the ideal. A creative balance would release the complacent from the restraints and provide relief from rebellion for the person seeking escape from all walls of life.

My decision to attend Clark University and pursue a college education at age sixty-eight provided relief from the wall of boredom which so quickly surrounds many people after retirement. The college environment and the classes, made up of students of varying ages, were stimulating and challenging for me, and the prospect of graduating some day encouraged me to look towards a brighter future.

Was this rediscovering spontaneity, as Emily was learning to do? A start, perhaps.

Originality

A rediscovery of originality plays a part in overcoming the walls of life, also. Originality, the dictionary says, is the *power to create new thoughts or combination of thoughts.* Probably one of the greatest challenges is to develop original ideas about aging or growing older and to find ways to cope with this time of life. As previously suggested, thoughts about aging only begin to surface at a point in life when a dramatic change takes place. Suddenly, or as it seems, the children are gone and a new way of living must be found. This is a distressing time—a time when one must surely rediscover originality in order to find productive work to do and leisure pastimes in which to engage. It is a time, also, to take stock of assets and liabilities and consider the options which are available.

Work, which has been a necessary part of life in some form since the beginning of history, must be considered as a healthy option for an activity throughout life. Work means different things to different people and in choosing work for the after-retirement years, it is important to concentrate on activities which are enjoyable and productive at the same time. Early childhood educators refer to children's play as their work. Mature adults, in the same way, can find rewarding work in cultivating a hobby.

Anna found a way to fill her later years with work which was, for her, both a hobby and a livelihood—enjoyable and productive.

Anna

At age seventy, Anna was a spry, lively lady who hadn't even considered retirement. The Great Depression and the death of her husband had made it necessary for her to provide a living for herself and her two children; almost her entire life was spent working at a variety of jobs.

In her late twenties and early thirties, she was not like a traditional wife and mother. Housework and cooking were no challenge for her; she wasn't interested in them. Convincing people to buy whatever she was selling was the challenge which she enjoyed.

Throughout her life, Anna was busy working, singing in choirs, and taking an active part in politics and community concerns, and so, when she was about seventy and clubs for older citizens were being organized, she attended one meeting and decided that she was not old enough to sit and drink tea and play games. She never did concede that she was old enough.

This spritely lady worked until she was eighty-two and probably never thought much about growing older until then. It was after this that she seemed to age—to become really old—with no work to do and little interest in working at home or in being at home every day. She was old. Her purpose for living had been taken from her. Work, her vocation and avocation, was her life. She loved selling things, whether it was hats, lamps, or natural foods. She could always present a convincing case for her goods.

Without the incentive to go to work daily, she lost interest in everything, even in living. It wasn't long before she was looking forward to whatever after-life was in store for her.

Anna was endowed with the qualities of spontaneity and originality and possessed a strength which I would wish to have to help me face any difficulties which may be part of my later years. It is not always easy to cultivate these qualities during the years after retirement. Women who have spent their adult lives caring for a home and family may find it more difficult to fill their time with rewarding activities than did Anna who continued at her usual work.

Anna was my mother.

Night Life

Opportunities for expressing originality sometimes appear in unexpected places. A shopping trip can become an open door to a new adventure such as *Night Life*. The sign over the counter read *Night Life*. That was an interesting concept since night life for us, my best friend Minor and I, had for many years consisted of getting the children into bed and collapsing into a chair with the newspaper. An occasional church supper or card game with friends provided some diversion away from the hum-drum everyday existence. So we thought we should investigate this *Night Life* that was being offered. Perhaps it would be an exciting new form of entertainment that two aging ladies could indulge in—hardly possible—but worth an inquiry.

Night Life did offer entertainment along with enrichment in the form of a multitude of activities, classes really, ranging from astrology to aerobics, powder puff mechanics to oil painting, wallpapering to skiing. We had already established ourselves in a gym class at the YWCA as exercise was one of the most important activities the retirement experts recommended. "Keep in good physical condition," they said," and you will feel better, stay young longer, and add years to your life." So we were working at that.

Our wallpapering ventures were well-known to our families—every room in the house was proof that we had been there with our paper and paste. They would never let us near the mechanics of the family car, driving it was concession enough. Oil painting—that was the most challenging offering as neither of us had ever been able to draw anything that was recognizable except possibly stick figures of people and houses with which to entertain the children during the Sunday sermon. Perhaps we would eventually be competition for Grandma Moses.

The next week, armed with easel, paints, brushes, and canvas, and wearing our smocks, we began our adventure as budding artists. It was like taking driving lessons—getting into the city traffic on the first lesson. No preliminaries—jump right in and get that landscape painted. That's the way we painted—learning as we worked. The colors were a mystery except for the primaries of red, blue, and yellow. Even those had many variations.

And perspective. That's very difficult. Making the lines come together at the vanishing point on the horizon. Just like in our lives, getting the right perspective on growing older, bringing all the parts together in order to have productive later years. Perspective in painting depends upon the position in which the artist is standing to observe her subject. So too, perspective on growing older is affected by our position as we look at our past experiences, our present condition, and what we hope for our future years.

Our experience with *Night Life* was enriching and provided us with a lasting hobby and an extra bonus of insight into the parallel between the artist's perspectives and our perspectives on growing older.

The Past

By the time I reached the age which is considered elderly, the past encompassed many years and provided me with a store of varied memories to call upon as a source of strength and enjoyment. As the magical age, assigned to those who are in the later years of life, approaches, memories of events, people, and experiences remembered become increasingly important.

What do I remember? Are some of the remembered happenings really stories which have been related to me? Do I remember more readily the happy times and relegate the sad, unpleasant events to a part of my memory that doesn't surface very often? Time, somehow, plays a part in lessening the impact of memories which are unpleasant and keeps near the surface those which make me happy. Do I consciously choose to recall the happenings which bring me pleasure and put into the recesses of my mind the hardships, frustrations, disagreements, and more serious occurrences of the past? I speak about the *good old days* and compare my memories of days past with the present which, probably because I am older, seems less exciting or pleasant. Again I am remembering the happy times.

Events of childhood: summer Sundays swimming and picnicking at Lake Park—the ride on the open trolley car; Thanksgiving train trips to visit grandparents in Providence—watching the ships, lights sparkling on the water, steam on the river in the evenings; struggling through waist-high snowdrifts to go to school; sliding and skiing in the park. And the Saturday movies and lunch at the mysterious Chinese restaurant upstairs on Main Street—the booths with beaded drapes around them and the waiter shuffling across the room with our orders of exotic foods with strange odors. All these were happy memories, but summer Sundays were the best.

Summer Sundays were different than Sundays the rest of the year. Summer Sundays belonged to Pa. The rest of the year Mother was in charge on Sunday. She was a church soloist and we spent Sundays at church, but when August came, the church closed for vacation. That was when Pa took over and changed our Sundays from long walks and long sermons to lazy days of fun and laughter. He loved those days—up early in the morning to cook breakfast before we started on the outing he had planned.

Usually, because Pa loved to swim, our destination was Lake Park on Lake Quinsigamond, a very popular swimming place, and we could get there on the trolley car. Trolley cars were a wonderful way to travel, especially if we were lucky enough to get on an open car. The motorman sat on his round stool-like seat at the front where he was in charge of keeping the car on the tracks. By clanging the bell with his foot, he kept the track clear of anything that might get in the way. When there was a long, flat stretch of road, he let the car go really fast, making it sway from side to side. The cool breeze swept past us and we clung to the wooden rail which kept us from falling into the street.

When the old stone tower at the top of the hill came into view, we knew we had reached our destination. It was a short walk to the lake and the large concrete bathhouse where we changed into our bathing suits. There was no sandy beach, so we sort of slithered over the edge of the wall into the water where Pa waited for us. He was a good swimmer and a good teacher and, with the help of our water-wings—rubber, balloon-like contraptions that stretched under our arms and appeared like wings on our backs—we tackled our swimming lesson.

A ball game was usually the afternoon diversion as we sat on the grass and relaxed after eating Pa's delicious lunch. Then, tired, sometimes sunburned, but always happy, we trudged back to the trolley for the trip home. Pa's Sunday was complete.

In a few short years Pa was no longer with us. I graduated from high school and, luckily, was able to find work. After three years, and with the Depression in full swing, I was married.

Jobs were almost non-existent and the company policy was that every woman who married must resign her job. Men were selling apples on the street corners or doughnuts door to door. There were no luxuries—six-room cold water flat, three rooms with furniture, stove heat. Electric washers, refrigerators, dishwashers, if available, were for the wealthy.

Our family grew over the next fifteen years to a total of seven people. Babies learning to walk and talk, their first school days, and then graduations and on to colleges. These were the war years also. Men leaving families to join the army or navy, food and gas rationing, air-raid alerts—all lights out, special black-out shades, and neighborhood men patrolling to make sure no lights could be seen—all a grim reality.

1954, and we were off to England to live for two years. Seven days on a beautiful ship crossing the Atlantic—a great adventure for a family which had never been far from Worcester.

Life was different in England. Shopping customs, heating methods, schools, and some foods were different. Even the language, although English, contained words which were unfamiliar to me. So, I learned a new English language.

The New English Language

Mrs. Morrison was coming to call. It was our second day in the sprawling, nine room house which was larger than our cottage at home but was sparsely furnished and had few modern conveniences. There was no washing machine, no central heating system, and shopping for food would be done daily, because the refrigerator was only the size of a large bread box.

Our family of four children, large by English standards, had already startled the quiet, sedate neighborhood. They played ball in the back garden and their shouts and whistles were the only sounds that could be heard. The little old lady next door peaked out from behind the curtains to see what the Americans, who had moved into the big house, were like.

The trunks were only half unpacked, the dishes were unwashed, and the fire was slowly dying in the tiny fireplace. Stephen, our two-year-old, was scampering wildly through the maze of hallways and rooms. Clearly, I was not ready for a visitor, especially Mrs. Morrison. Mrs. Morrison was the wife of the Manager, and although she was a native Scot, she conformed to the proprieties of the upper-class English lady. Promptly at two o'clock she arrived dressed in a mauve tweed suit and wearing a purple felt hat; she was carrying her gloves and purse. When the customary greetings and introductions were over and

Stephen had found a hiding place, at least for a few minutes, we went into the living room. It was a long room with a small fireplace at one end and large glass doors overlooking the rose garden. Two large wing chairs, designed to keep the drafts away from the occupants, were beside the fire, which was now providing a little heat for the very chilly room.

While enjoying freshly brewed tea and cookies, we continued our conversation which turned out to be my indoctrination into the whys and wherefores of obtaining food to feed my husband and children. It was a strange thing about coming to live in England. I expected that—it being an English-speaking country—language and customs would be the same as at home. Not so, I found, as Mrs. Morrison presented her list of how and where to buy food.

"You most certainly must have a butcher and greengrocer," she said, "who come to the house and take your orders and deliver the food to the house. My butcher has absolutely the best meat. His mince is the finest in town, and I know you will like his rashers of gammon. I'll order some for you and send my greengrocer over to see you when he comes on Tuesday." I agreed to her arrangements, but the language was puzzling me— greengrocer, mince, rashers, gammon. I wasn't quite sure what we would be eating.

Already we had learned a new automobile language. *Boot* for trunk, *bonnet* for hood, *windscreen* for windshield, *hooter* for horn, tire was spelled with a y; we bought petrol not gas, and kept to the left at the roundabouts. Now, here was a new food language I had to deal with.

Mrs. Morrison finished her tea, and, obviously distressed by Stephen's antics, said her polite goodbyes and left.

On Tuesday morning, as I was again struggling to coax the big lumps of coal to light and give us some heat, the bell sounded a quick, tingling ring, accompanied by the happy whistling of whoever stood outside.

"Good morning, Love," he said, as I opened the door. "I'm the greengrocer. Mrs. Morrison said you would like to see me today."

Very familiar, I thought, calling me *Love* the first time he saw me. Maybe that's the way Englishmen were, although they had a reputation of being very quiet and reserved.

He was a tall, thin man with happy, sparkling eyes, a quick smile, and the typical ruddy complexion of an Englishman who spends most of his time outdoors in the damp, cool weather. His black beret was tipped on the side of his head and he wore a gray wool sweater, heavy boots, and narrow, shiny black pants. Over his shoulder he carried his money bag, a large, leather pouch which held the assorted English coins—pence, shillings, half-crowns, and the paper pounds. More new language!

"And what is it you would like today, Love?" he asked. "I have sprouts, marrow, beetroot, potatoes, carrots, and squash."

Not wanting to appear too ignorant and assuming the sprouts must be brussel sprouts and the beetroot must be beets, I ordered some of each along with potatoes and carrots. At least I couldn't go wrong on those. Still not sure about the marrow and the squash—was it butternut, summer or blue hubbard—I asked to see them. We went out to his van and I saw what looked like a zucchini squash.

"Oh," he said. "that's marrow. Now would you like lemon or orange squash?

How did I know? Lemon seemed to be a good choice. Maybe that was summer squash.

"Yes, Love, I hope you will like this English squash," he said, as he handed me a bottle of lemon-colored liquid which resembled lemonade.

Somewhat abashed, I picked up my basket of vegetables and bottle of squash, paid him the pounds, shillings, and pence he asked for and returned to the kitchen. I was right about the beetroot, anyway; they were beets with one difference—he had already cooked them.

Another lesson learned. The butcher would be next with his mince and rashers of gammon. He arrived the same afternoon. The bell rang slowly and deliberately and I opened the door to a very serious gentleman dressed in a long white butcher's coat and a small English tweed cap Very quietly he handed me the packages of meat, almost as if they were an offering to the gods. They were, indeed, rather special since meat was still rationed and we were very lucky to be able to get any.

31

Once again I offered my assorted English currency, still not quite sure what any of it was worth. I was impatient to discover just what we would be eating for dinner and quickly unwrapped the outer paper—part of an old newspaper—then the inside wrapping, to discover I had two pounds of the best hamburg and a pound of sliced bacon. The mystery of mince and rashers of gammon was solved.

This was not the end of my English language education. I learned about sugar, at least four kinds—demararra, castor, icing, granulated; lemon cheese which wasn't cheese at all but a lemon filling; Victoria sandwich which wasn't a sandwich but a layer cake; and biscuits which were really cookies.

Mince, squash, rashers, and gammon—a good beginning to my new English vocabulary. Enough lessons for one day. I went back to the unpacking and to Stephen, wherever he was.

There would be other trips, living in strange countries—Germany, Korea, and Poland. Then we would be home again. Each time our memories were safely stored away for blue Mondays or story time with Sarah, Jeannie, and Carrie.

Foundations and Faith

From early childhood, foundations allow us to build strong character with enduring qualities. These are the foundations on which people in their later years depend. The work we have done, our relations with family and friends, our ability to meet disappointments and misfortunes with courage, and the development of a lasting faith are part of the foundations which we will use to carry us through the present and future.

To strengthen these foundations and to develop a lasting faith, it was necessary for me, through the years, to consider my religious training and to do considerable pondering and searching, reading and analyzing, in order to discover the difference between facts presented to me and my own perception of religious truths and how it all fit together for me as an individual. What did I believe?

Organized religion can become very complicated and oftentimes very confusing, with a variety of trappings which, for me, had to be set aside in order to get to a basic belief and faith. I needed to find what my perception of God was as an influence in my life. This had to be a belief in a power working within me—the Holy Spirit, if you will— which provided strength, comfort, and relative peace and was an inspiration for relating to family, friends, and the community.

The thirty years during which my family was growing presented problems and crises as well as happy times. These were the years when I needed to be strong in order to cope with the stresses and strains of raising a large family. Parents and friends gave advice, but finally, I had to find solutions within myself. To do that, I needed a strong faith.

Professor Jerome Ellison considers spiritual growth a necessary concern for people in the later years of life. He claims,

> *Mature people, those who have finished acquiring material goods, offspring, club memberships, should and must, if life is to have continued meaning, work for internal growth. It is the internal work, the spiritual growing with which the mature man and woman must be concerned.*

This internal work, the spiritual growing which Ellison deems necessary for mature adults to cultivate, becomes a part of achieving the new fulfillment of life as suggested by Tournier.

Faith and belief in a power greater than man strengthens as a person passes through the experiences of adulthood. Hardships, disappointments, and sorrows are met and overcome with greater ease by a person who has developed an inner strength through faith and belief in this unseen power. Each encounter that is successfully overcome strengthens belief in self and in God and produces confidence and an increased faith in dealing with future situations.

The Bible offers inspiration, strength, and comfort and gives direction to our lives. The Psalms speak to every condition of man. The First psalm describes the way of life necessary for happiness. Psalm 23 gives comfort and assurance in time of trouble and Psalm 121 offers strength and help in time of need.

Direction for our lives comes from many parts of this most popular book:

> *What does the Lord require of you but to do justice, love mercy, and walk humbly with your God* (Micah 6:8).

And reinforcing this quotation:

> *Love your neighbor as yourself* (Matthew 7:12).

The Golden Rule,

> *So whatever you wish that men would do to you, do so to them* (Matthew 7:12),

and the Ten Commandments provide further direction. When the stress and rush of the world overwhelm us, the admonition,

> *Be still and know that I am God* (Psalm 46),

If heeded, becomes a calming influence on our lives.

Our thoughts are directed by the advice:

> *Finally, brethren, whatever is true, whatever is honorable, whatever is just, whatever is pure, whatever is lovely, whatever is gracious, if there is*

any excellence, if there is anything worthy of praise, think about these things (Philippians 4:8).

And the Psalmist, contemplating the passage of time, prays:

Do not cast me off in the time of old age, forsake me not when my strength is spent (Psalms 71:9).

Dr. Bortz describes the benefits of a religious faith when he says, "A deep religious faith, whatever its form, matured throughout a lifetime, furnishes the aged person with a quiet, serene, and undemanding understanding."

I believe that my life has been enriched by the faith I have acquired and I am grateful for the foundations laid in the past which have helped me endure through the years.

The Present: Retirement

Retirement, that long anticipated time of relief from work and responsibility; time for leisure activities, travel and relaxation; time to do whatever comes to mind, is upon us. However, we are finding that leisure is fine for a short time, but complete absence of responsibility and meaningful work or activities produces boredom and frustration for us.

On reaching the time of retirement, one establishes a new routine and makes adjustments to accommodate this new pattern of living. These adjustments are more drastic for a person who has worked all his or her life in a productive job and whose time has been regulated by others than for a person who has always worked at home and organized his or her own time around household duties and family responsibilities. The stay-at-home person has to find ways of working with another person in the house all day. He or she has to use time in new ways, working around the schedule of the other person.

I find that as circumstances change for me and less and less is required of me, new challenges take the place of previous commitments and I use my time differently. Family demands are diminished and it is easy to change plans and activities. Opportunities for volunteer service abound, while more and more part-time work is available to older people.

Present-day life for the elderly is, in many ways and for most people, more comfortable than it ever was in the past. Government agencies have concentrated on providing housing, food subsidies, Social Security, medical care, recreation, and other benefits for the older citizens so that they may maintain a good quality of life. Housing developments provide safe, low-cost living for older people who are unable to cope with the care of their own homes. These complexes become an active community, some being almost self-contained units with shopping facilities and medical clinics within the grounds. They provide companionship and offer security and relief from the many cares of maintaining a large house.

This type of housing, however, has some disadvantages. In recent years, the elderly have become increasingly a segregated minority, living in ghetto-like communities of old people. Some older people prefer to live separated from young people and children after their own families are grown. The more affluent move to golden-age developments in Florida or Arizona, while those who cannot afford this luxury living might become residents of high-rise buildings devoted exclusively to the elderly.

Families formerly lived close together with grandparents very often living with the younger generations. Today they are separated. Children and grandchildren no longer live in the same neighborhood with grandparents. Many children are unfamiliar with even one older person and this widens the gap between young and old. In the December, 1981, issue of *Gerontology,* Bronfenbrenner is quoted as saying, as early as 1970, that:

> *If the current trend persists, if the institutions of our society continue to remove parents, other adults, … from active participation in the lives of our children, and if the resulting vacuum is filled by the age-segregated peer group, we can anticipate increased alienation, indifference, antagonism and violence on the part of the younger generation in all segments of our society.*

It is encouraging to note that some housing developments are being built which allow families with children, the elderly, and the handicapped to share the available apartments.

But stereotypes associated with aging have developed because of this segregation of ages. These stereotypes are expressed by society which says that there is a chronological age at which people become unfit for productive work, that the elderly are unable to care for themselves, are to be pitied, have lost their memories, are too feeble to conduct their own affairs, and that all old people are the same.   Fischer says that when these stereotypes persist American becomes a closed society for the aged.

As in any age group there are those who society must care for or who must have assistance in caring for themselves, but the majority of aging adults believe that they are as self-sufficient as any other segment of the population. Cicero, in his famous treatise, said,

> *Again, there is no fixed borderline for old age and you are making a good and proper use of it as long as you can satisfy the call of duty and disregard death. The result of this is, that old age is even more confident and courageous than youth.*

In recent years, an emphasis has been placed on youth and this has resulted in an early discard of older people. A shift in this idea becomes necessary when we consider the declining birthrate and the extended longevity brought about by advanced medical care and an increased awareness of the need for good health and dietary habits throughout life. Fischer presents statistics which show that the elderly part of the population, those over sixty-five, grew from less than two percent in the 1800s to ten percent in 1970. He also points out that only one American out of five survived to the age of seventy in 1750 and that by 1970, four out of five were reaching that age.

The aging process does leave its mark on people of all ages, but the ambition of every older person who wishes to live a full and rewarding life should be to live with continued enthusiasm, making no excuses for being older. Many have accepted the role assigned to them by television, newspapers, and advertising and believe that, because they are perceived in a particular way, they must live as they are seen. This leads to an early decline in enthusiasm, curiosity, and interest in continued growth.

As early as age fifty, there are those who make excuses about their age such as when they claim: *My memory isn't what it used to be.* There is probably some loss in ability to remember, but I would ask, "Could you always remember things when you were younger?" Young people forget things, too. Are we allowing our powers to become dull from lack of effort or use? Cicero's answer would be:

> But it is said, memory dwindles. No doubt, unless you keep it in practice, or if you happen to be somewhat dull by nature .... Old men retain their intellects well enough, if only they keep their minds active and fully employed.

Then we hear the *at my age* excuse whenever something happens which requires a reason for certain behavior. Excuses are no substitute for honest endeavors to continue to use and exercise all our faculties.

I consider my present circumstances and try to bring into perspective my outlook on aging. The present is a good time for me. I have good health, a comfortable home, a loving family and friends to be with, and an adequate income. I am able to look at aging in a much different way than does someone who is poor, lonely and physically disabled. Aging, from my present position seems no different than it did in the past. I spend little time concentrating on how old I am and continue to plan for a good future.

The question, I believe, is how my perspectives of the past and present will blend with my vision of the future to produce a happy, fulfilling life for my later years.

The Future

The future, at any age, is a vast unknown. Nothing is sure except that time will continue to pass and the future will always be there for someone. As I look towards the future and consider the public image of growing older, it is as if the growing has stopped and the goal has been reached. There's no further to go—no growing to do.

The fashion designers concentrate on styles for young people, hairdressers have only one style for the female senior citizen, television ads present the elderly women in arthritis or wrinkle-erasing ads. Yet there are many who have reached this magical age who still feel a need to continue to grow and learn and enjoy life as younger people do. Each age presents problems, and a plethora of magazines is available to help cope with these problems— *Parents* for the child-rearing ages; *Dynamic Years* for the mid-life person, *Modern Maturity* for the older adult, and others, all adding to the categorization of people into age-related groups.

Young, middle-aged, old. Where is the division? Is it a matter of passing of time, chronological age, adding years? Or is it, more clearly, a matter of state of mind; a philosophy of living; a way of looking at life with a long-range view and hope for many productive years; a plan for the future which is positive; a growing experience until life is finished at whatever age? It is inevitable that the ultimate climax of life is old age and finally death. However, to attain old age does not mean to stop living but to continue life into a new phase which can be as rich and rewarding as any other period of life.

My future depends upon what I have put into the past and the present and how I look at the coming years. I can only speculate from a position of strength and hope as to what the future holds for me. As the artist uses his training and experience on which to build when creating his artistic work, so I must use my past experiences and accumulation of knowledge to influence my future. The artist knows that he must have dark areas on his canvas in order to make the lights more brilliant. Similarly, I know from past experience that there will be dark times in my future—discouragement, illness, sadness—but that light, happy times, good health, love of family and friends will be brighter when projected against the dark times.

As I grow older, my life will be enriched if I learn to see more clearly the world and the variety of experiences available to me. Again, I turn to the artist who learns how to see every part of a picture—color variations, shapes of clouds and trees, distance and close-up, facial expressions, individual parts of flowers, brilliance of sunrise and sunset, and the unending motion of the sea—in order to capture the beauty of nature and man on the canvas.

Looking more closely, I see new ways to continue to grow and learn, and if I look with sharper vision, seeing the new possibilities of growth, I realize that my world teems with opportunities. I widen my horizons and leave behind the narrow view of life. If I see and understand myself better, acknowledging weaknesses and strengths and searching for ways to overcome the weaknesses and to fortify the strengths, a new view of my remaining years is apparent.

Family and friends appear in a new light when seen through my artist's eyes. Their pleasing qualities are discovered and emphasized and they become part of a store of strengths gathered together for support. It is easy in later years to become disgruntled and pessimistic and see only the unlikeable characteristics in others. A more optimistic attitude brings a happier outlook for the future.

If we have lived an active life with an optimistic attitude toward aging, our future as older citizens should continue to be active and optimistic. Maurois has said,

> To love the good in people around me and to avoid the wicked, to enjoy my good fortune and to bear my ill, and to remember to forget, that has been my optimism. It has helped me to live. May it help you, too.

A fitting philosophy for any age, but especially for the later years of life.

The pendulum is slowly swinging. Attitudes are changing once more. The present generation of elderly is presenting a new image of growing old. They are continuing to grow in spite of their age and are looking to a future which will offer them a full life if they make the right choices. Choices are never easy to make, but for the aging a wider range is available for those who are physically and mentally able and have the desire to remain active in their later years.

Society is beginning to understand that the elderly have been neglected in the past and adjustments are being made to accommodate their needs. Medical schools now require a course in geriatrics to enable young physicians to recognize the medical needs of older patients. Colleges are encouraging those over sixty to return to school and many are taking advantage of the opportunity for further education. Mandatory retirement at age sixty-five is no longer a requirement for workers and some older employees are choosing to remain at work—an open choice now. The elderly are becoming a strong lobby to influence the legislators as they make decisions concerning older citizens. Life is, indeed, better for the present generation of older people and their future appears brighter than ever before.

Fischer, in writing about the future of the aging population in America, proposes that the work ethic should not be the only ethical belief which is important to society. He suggests other ethical structures—ethics of being, for instance, such as an ethic of experience, of perception, of participation, of feeling, of sharing, of enduring, or an ethic of simply surviving. He believes that a person should be able to choose which ethic he wishes to adopt and challenges the American humanists to study the ethical variety of life in order to learn how strong and broad the ethical possibilities of life are.

However you try to understand it or think about it and whatever ethical focus you choose to live by, aging is art and aging *is* an art. Look around you. Look at the colors, the sizes, the shapes, all the horizons, all the possibilities. And then paint your glorious roadmap to the future in brilliant Technicolor. I, for one, plan to use Maurois' proposition as the compass to my senior trail:

> *Old age is far more than white hair, wrinkles, the feeling that it is too late and the game finished, that the stage belongs to the rising generations. The true evil is not the weakening of the body, but the indifference of the soul.*

Conversation 2

Another year, another summer. Sarah is clambering over the rocks once more. She is eight years old now, and I, too, have added another year. We look across to the lighthouse. The beacon flashes out over the ocean as it has

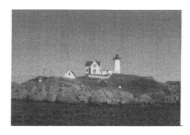

for so many years. The sea, too, is unchanged. Waves continue to crash against the rocks; the sun appears each day on the eastern horizon, glistening on the water, and

sets, in a blaze of gold and red, in the West; gulls screech and cry as they glide above the waves, dive down for the elusive fish, then swoop high into the air—all evidence of the dependability of nature. The pessimistic news of the world seems remote and we are transported for a short time into the calm and carefree world.

"Grandma, there's a ship out there. I wonder where it is going," Sarah ponders.

"Maybe we can guess," I reply, and as we look toward the ship on the horizon, we think of all the places it might travel to—England, France, Africa, India, even around the world.

So it is with my remaining years. I look to the horizon of my life and imagine the things I can do, places I can go, friendships I can nurture, and family I can love. The passing of the seasons hasn't significantly changed my feelings and attitudes about growing older. It is a good time!

Grow old along with me!
The best is yet to be.
The last of life, for which the first was made:
Our times are in his hand
Who saith, "A whole I planned;
Youth shows but half; trust God: see all, nor be afraid!"

Robert Browning in *Rabbi Ben Ezra*

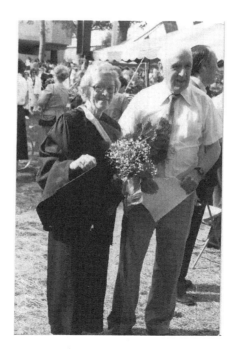

List of Sources

Bortz, E.L. (1963). *Creative aging.* New York, New York: MacMillan Company.
(pages 162-167; 178-179)

Cicero, M.T. (40 B.C.). Trans. by W. Melmoth. On old age. In C.W. Elliot (Ed.). (1909). *The Harvard classics.* New York, NY: P.F. Collier & Son.
(pages 53; 59; 72)

Davis, R.H. (1981, Dec-Jan). Intergenerational relationships. *Gerontologist.*
(page 568)

Downs, H. (1978-1979, Dec-Jan.). How I plan to celebrate my 100th birthday. *Modern Maturity.*
(pages 39-40)

Ellison, J. (1975, Oct-Nov). Man with a message. *Modern Maturity.*
(page 67)

Fischer, D. H. (1977). *Growing old in America.* New York, NY: Oxford University Press.
(pages 35; 114; 116; 118-119; 217-219)

Kaasa, O. J. (1981-1982, Dec-Jan). How to give meaning to your life. *Modern Maturity.* (page 4)

Maurois, A. *Letters to an unknown lady.* http://www.brainyquote.com/quotes/quotes/a/andremauro158002.html

Tournier, P. (1981-1982, Dec-Jan). Learning to grow old. *Modern Maturity.* (page 4)

Also by Mabel Monks:

On the Water in *Reflections* (Volume I) (2005). York, Maine: Sentry Hill Writers

Summer's End in *Reflections* (Volume I) (2005). York, Maine: Sentry Hill Writers

Elbridge Boyden, Architect: His Life and Work, 1810-1898. (1989). Database: Worldcat.org

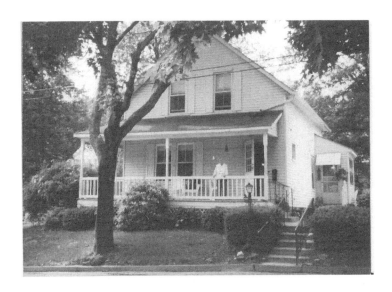

20585040R00041

Made in the USA
Middletown, DE
01 June 2015